Stress Management & Learning Techniques
For Medical Students,
Doctors & Dentists.

A compilation of validated stress management techniques
and learning techniques for Medical Students, Doctors &
Dentists, to prevent burnout and enable us to thrive in our
medical careers.

Dr. Pritam Biswas MBBS, MD.

Dedication

To my parents and little sister, who continue to inspire me.

Contents

Stress Management Techniques

Learning Techniques

Stress Management Techniques

Stress Management Techniques

There is a belief in the myth that, "the experience of stress is unavoidable and is an accomplice to our life pursuits and challenges. Avoiding it would make us unproductive and inefficient". Optimum stress is necessary in our lives; however the subjective effect it has on your thoughts, mood, physiology and behavior is definitely not a necessity.

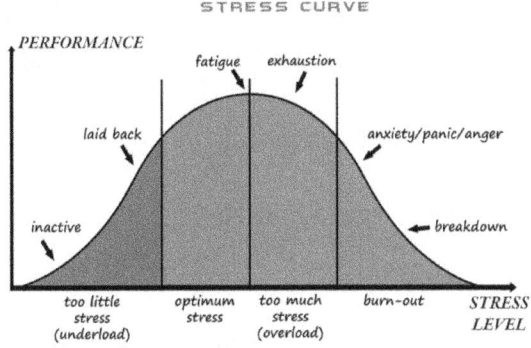

STRESS CURVE

The goal of this book is not to eliminate stress, but to change your perception of it, such that it has no effect to take over your life. In this way we can pursue our challenges, accomplish more and become resilient professionals.

As a child, when learning to ride a bicycle we get knocked over several times, however over time you excel at it. Likewise, let us start learning the techniques of stress management down the road towards resilience.

Chapter 1

"Clarifying Personal Values"- Find your Fuel for life

As medical professionals, often we sail through the difficult hectic days, with utmost ease functioning at full throttle. Yet some days are long arduous and take a toll on us .

So what makes the difference?

It is the subconscious knowledge of *"Why we do, what we do?"*

Yes, it's the simple understanding of what we want out of life. What ideals/values we look up to and who we want to be known as.

Example

After a hectic long shift at the hospital after returning home, your family has decided to go shopping and need you to drive them to the mall. At this point of time your only wish is to get some rest and unwind.

Either you grumble about having to drive in traffic .Drive them there and complain all the way and make the experience for you and them a negative unpleasant one .

Or

You drive them, to make them happy and yet furiously annoyed within.

Either ways there is a lot of negativity around this, situations like these that leads to subconscious buildup of stress gradually over time.

So how do we handle this?
Answer the question, *"Why we do, what we do?"*

A **simple mental clarification** on your ideals/values is required.

Hypothetically one of your ideals being *To be caring and protective towards your family. (A good son/daughter/spouse / parent)*

Is all it takes to make the stresses that daily life throw at us more bearable and convert them into opportunities to achieving our ideals/values.

Whether is filling out tedious paperwork and documentation in the hospital or driving in rush hour to be on time, dealing with difficult colleagues, patients, professors. All these mindless mundane activities though seemingly innocuous, contribute to a lot of subconscious buildup of stress.

A simple clarification of one's personal ideals , can mitigate the mundane everyday work and events from leading to stress .

Now one may confuse ideals with goals they are two very different things. Ideals are the "why" we set certain goals for ourselves.

Step One: Answer the "WHY?

E.g.

You were looking forward to a difficult set of exams; this could be a potential source of a lot of chronic stress. As we all know going after certain dreams, comes with their set of hurdles. There may be time delays, financial emergencies, pessimism of peers with comments of "that's too difficult" or "are you sure your capable of that?" ,technical difficulties , personal problems, booked out travel routes, innumerable unforeseen circumstances . As well as innocuous mundane daily routines like traffic jams , long lines at your supermarkets, usurping your valuable time which can lead to a built up of stress.

The best way to go about it would be find out your inner thoughts of why are you are going to take these particular set of exams .You may rationalize and come up with different reasons," that they may give you more respect ", "they would help your career" or a common explanation like "every other doctor is doing it too, so I will do it as well " or " I will be financially more secure ". So whatever the reasons may be, you need to look into your personal ideals/values.

Your ideals/values are your personal energy; they reflect your passion and your spirit. You need to capitalize on it, to go forth into manifesting your dreams, surviving the various stressors that brings about.

Ideals/Values Clarification

Domain	List of ideals
Education 1.Specialist Exams " subject X "	1. To be an authority on subject X 2. To make my family proud of me 3. To be respected among peers, subordinates, seniors, patients.

We as medical professionals have been there, done that. Countless years of education, hundreds of sleepless nights, assimilating pathophysiology s of hundreds of medical conditions .So you might say "This is what I do all the time, how do you think I survived in medicine this long?"

Well it's not all about "surviving"

A formal reaffirmation of your ideals/values, not only lets you "survive ", but it helps you connect with your passion to "thrive ". You can utilize them to overcome any of the daily stressors or mindless mundane work that may dwindle your energies and dominate your life. Enumerate them mentally or say them aloud if you're alone (unless your going for the mad scientist image). The point being it brings these thoughts to the forefront of your mind set and gives you the energy to "thrive " and not just be on survival mode.

Exercise 1

Take a few minutes out to fill in the table below:

Domain	List of Ideals/Values.
Personal life	
Work life	
Recreation	
Health (Physical/mental)	
Social life	
Other domains	

Once you filled out the table, you are now armed with your personal "fuel" to tide over any stressful situation that life may bring to you in any domain.

Chapter 2

Introduction to Emotional Management

Our emotional re-activity can either empower or dis-empower the effect of chronic stress.

We generalize emotions either into "good" or bad based on how they make is feel, but on the contrary all emotions serve a purpose. They represent raw untamed forces of our sub consciousness, and we can utilize them as tools to mitigate the effects of chronic stress.

There are no good or bad emotions it's all about the perspective that we perceive them to be.

For example

Emotion	Ideal utilization
Positive emotions happiness joy awe gratefulness	Expansive and broadens thought process and helps in expansive thinking. Exploration of interests , Ambitions Respect, curiosity, leadership Contribution, giving
Negative emotions anger sadness irritability discontent jealously boredom	Narrows focuses thought process and helps in problem solving , making decisions putting an end to a stressor instigating change competitiveness creative ideas

So these hold great power within them, but unfortunately being products of 10 million years of evolution has not given us an edge in managing these primeval forces.

We remain or enthusiastically remain slaves to them and go through our lives in blindly serving them. All the things we do in life, work, studies, shopping, cooking stem from the need to pacify emotions, primeval emotions of happiness, joy.

So does that mean we need to demonize the negative emotions?

No, they too serve great purpose, in self-preservation in problem solving and instigating change in our lives.

The Following chapters deal with techniques to:

Manage Negative Emotions

The Practice of Positive Emotions

Chapter 3

Managing Negative emotions

Technique 1

Identification, labeling and Quantification of emotion

This technique has been verified by cognitive psychologists, The act of intentional awareness of the feeling that you experience, labeling it as a specific emotion (anger, sadness, boredom, nervousness, anxiety etc.) helps in viewing the sensation objectively from a conscious rational mind and not subjectively as a feeling that is controlling you and your mindset.

Going a step further to rate it on a scale (0-10) involves thinking and rational mind, this is known to decrease the intensity and effect of the emotion.

Example: When pain scales are used in succession on patients, the subjective intensity is known to decrease.

In a hypothetical scenario:

" You have spent a 12 hour shift in the hospital and about to hand over charge to the next doctor, when you are called in ,as there the is an issue in the wards with one of your patients. On arriving at patients bed, the patients attendant is the one demanding to see the doctor. The relative is emotionally upset and being from the medical fraternity poses some interrogative questions to you regarding the treatment and irrationally hurls accusations of negligence and questions your expertise. Going so far, as to demand another physician.

A situation like this can elicit a lot of lot of different emotions anger, sadness and defensiveness.

As health care professionals we suppress the emotion and try our best to handle this professionally or act out irrationally at times displaying negative responses that we regret at a later point in time.

So what is the right thing to do?

Now, both these responses do not help us .Suppression of emotion, leads to a chronic build up over time. Your psyche wants you to validate what it experiences.

Conversely reacting to the situation will worsen the problem to a further extent.

The answer - Experience it, Objectively identify it, label it and quantify it and finally channelize it.

Step 1

Observe the feeling, Identify it and do not suppress it or push it away.

Step 2

Give the emotion a specific name

Step 3

Rate it on a scale of 0-10

These 3 steps segregate the emotion as an entity and bring in your reasoning into the process of your perception.

Step 4

Know that this emotion or feeling is separate from, who you are as a person. "You are not your emotion", you have our own set of ideals and values to live by.

Cognitive Psychologists have systematically prove that the above technique reduces the intensity of these emotions.

Technique 2

Relaxation response through guided imagery and progressive muscle relaxation.

It has been shown that we can consciously pay attention to only one thing at a time, this might surprise multitaskers with disbelief. However, our ability to quickly shift between tasks and thoughts of different subjects very rapidly gives us the illusion of multitasking.

We can utilize this knowledge effectively when managing stress, by disengaging from negative emotions and thoughts that activate the stress response and shift our awareness to positive thoughts and emotions that bring about a relaxation response.

Experiments have demonstrated that the mind reacts to experiences, irrespective if it's real or imagined, it cannot tell the difference.

When watching a horror or an action movie, does bring about physiological changes like rise in blood pressure apart from the subjective emotional response.

In an experiment done with Olympic athletes and swimmers. These swimmers were monitored with myographs, EEG, BP and heart rate Monitors. They were then asked to visualize performing their activity with closed eyes. Following which the monitors recorded synchronous firing of groups of muscles involved in swimming with alternate firing of each limb and a raise in blood pressure and respiratory rate.

The mind cannot tell the difference between real or imaginary, its only our thinking patterns that acts as a filter.

When we are exposed to chronic stress our thinking patterns are selectively narrowed down. We tend to view things in a negative light. Cynicism, pessimism are the birth child of chronic negative thinking.

If the mind cannot tell the difference between real and imaginary, this can be used to our advantage in our quest towards managing stress.

Technique:

Step 1

Schedule 5 to 10 minutes a day for guided imagery and progressive muscle relaxation

Step 2

Seat yourself or lie down, take long deep slow breaths.

Step 3

Be aware of the sensations in your body, your emotions (any anxiety stresses fears)and be aware of the muscle tension in the body .

Step 4

Start the process of relaxation from the toes, relax all the muscles gradually from toes to ankles and ascend gradually intentionally relaxing each muscle. Gently relax the muscles of the claves, thigh's, hips and abdomen, chest arms and fingers .Taking a few seconds at each spot to ensure that the muscles are relaxed in a slow gradual process

It's very important to take your time in relaxing the muscles of the neck, jaw muscles of the face and the eyelids and scalp.

Scan your body now from head to toe and release any tension left

Step 5

As you lie motionless, breathing deeply and slowly, acknowledge that you have both negative and positive thoughts and choose to scale up the positive ones and fill your awareness with feeling good.

The goal here is to build a mental image that involves the perception from all the physical senses.

Step 6.

Imagine yourself in a place of peace and tranquility, preferably a picturesque beach. Engage all senses in your imagination.

Feel the warm sunlight and cool air the grainy soft sand beneath your feet, the salty smell of the ocean, the sounds of the waves and the birds. Make the picture and experience as real and vivid as possible. Bask in this state for as long as you have time.

Step 7

Open your eyes stretch and carry on with your day.

We doctors can be quite skeptical on these techniques, they have had significant results on stress levels in cancer patients and even shown to decrease levels of anxiety and in hypertensives have decreased blood pressure on continued practice .

This technique is the opposite of sleeping, as when you are asleep there is dimming of mental faculties. However guided imagery is an active process where you are alert and mentally experiencing a situation which sets of a relaxation response(or as we know the parasympathetic system). Calming the mind and making us more effective and resilient to face the day ahead.

Technique 3

Self-soothing

Self-soothing or self-care techniques are known to be a great way to relieve stress. While social support from family and friends, can be the best mechanism they are not always readily available thus appropriate awareness of the use of self-soothing is essential to build resilience and to thrive even in difficult circumstances.

The goal of self-soothing is to engage all 5 senses and involve the mind in uplifting activity

How do time strapped medics take time to achieve this?

Develop your own personalized box of self-soothing activities that uplift each of the 5 senses on a daily basis, that is available to you in your surroundings.

1. Whether it is a walk around your university campus/hospital for a few minutes of quiet and calm
2. Savoring your cup of tea/ coffee by yourself for a few minutes .
3. Listening to your favorite music for a few minutes.

You need to develop your own go to that you can incorporate in your daily schedule.This is mandatory on a daily basis to take the edge of the stresses of the day, reserve a few minutes for yourself.

Chapter 4

The Practice of Positive Emotion

Evidence based studies have shown the effectiveness of raising and maintaining a positive mindset in stress reduction.

The most effective way to do this is the ***Practice of gratitude***

Independent studies have demonstrated its effectiveness on mood (increased experience of happiness, optimism joyfulness), as well as physiological changes (better subjective quality of sleep and fewer illnesses and improvement of immunity), improved mental faculties (improved problem solving) and improved social wellbeing (fostering interpersonal connections).

Practice of gratitude

Gratitude is the appreciation of what is valuable and meaningful to oneself and is a state of being thankful and appreciative

1. Counting your blessing in your free time or during a break, thinking about the good in your life and what you are happy to have . Whether it's your family, friends or a meal that you have . Gratitude creates

sense abundance and changes your perspective on your current life situation and events. This feeling of abundance creates a sense of completeness which helps you view your current wants, dreams, desires and needs as a endeavor to greater happiness and not as scarcity in your life.

2. Intentionaly practice and visualize, knowing that you are already in a place of content and happiness and that you have so much that you are already grateful for. This can be practiced while doing mundane activities such as when you are in the shower or when your cooking or during the commute to work and during your daily chores . If time permits, perhaps maintain a diary or a smartphone note app.

3. When confronted with a negative situation or a negative emotion, be grateful for it. As it is giving you something very important, a learning experience an opportunity to take corrective action for the future, or knowledge of what behaviors in yourself you need to modify.

Ask yourself questions:

"What can I learn from this ?"
"How do I deal with this situation ?"
"How to plan ahead the next time around?"
Etc

Finding the silver lining, and being grateful for it helps you learn and become resilient to negative situations

4. Display gratitude towards others, with a simple 'thank you' with honesty or a simple appreciation , however do not resort to flattery.

   "In giving positive emotions to others we lift up our own positive state of mind"

   You can be creative, simple thank you notes or messages to a visit of people you are grateful to.

5. Except your compliments
   When someone says thank you, acknowledge their need to tell you about how grateful they are. Do not

brush it aside, as its devaluing their gratitude as well as disrespecting yourself, as you need to accept the respect that you deserve

Accepting thanks allows you to build your self-esteem, confidence and this in turn creates a positive mindset.

Achieving a "Flow" State.

This state is described by individuals who become absorbed and completely involved in an activity, whether it be playing chess, exercise, cooking, studying a subject or during giving a presentation. They experience a subjective feeling called the "flow state" of complete engrossment.

The flow state is a feeling movement in time in which the person is in control of his/her actions and in which there is little distinction between self and activity that he is doing while being oblivious of time, stimulus or response.

This merging of action and awareness, basically total and complete focus on an activity is a pleasurable feeling that most people have experienced with varied activities of interest. It is a motivator for the interests and pursuits in life as well as a perfect way to generate positive emotion and emotional balance.

Find activities that are of interest to you and develop this feeling of absolute attention to experience flow on a regular basis .

Chapter 5

Mindfulness Based Stress Reduction Practices

Reconnecting with the 'now'

Mindfulness based practices, though having roots in eastern Indian and Tibetan philosophy, has gathered great attention over the last decade as cognitive psychologists and neurologists have extensively studied the impacts of these practices on brain function of subjects and effect on patients. There are evidences of improved concentration, improved mental function, improvement of chronic diseases and stress related disorders. There are nearly 700 publications on mindfulness based practices that appear in pub med every year they have even been incorporated into the various health systems of different countries. As members of the medical community what stops us from applying this in our own lies. It the misconception, that these practices take time and as a medical student or a physician they are variety of time consuming activities in our busy schedule. In the course of this chapter we shall mention a handful of simple techniques which can be applied in our daily schedule.

What is mindlessness?

To understand the Mindfulness Based Practice one must first understand what is 'mindlessness'. Mindlessness can be described as our monkey brain due to years of evolution in helping us maintain homeostasis. It is having reactive thoughts to a particular situation, dwelling on random thoughts and letting it affect us emotionally, the constant thoughts of the future or past experiences or it is simply living on auto pilot going about daily activities without giving it much thought

E.g. going through the daily morning routine of showering, eating breakfast and getting ready, commuting and not realizing how automatic the process is. That sudden realization of awakening when you reach your workplace and not having a memory of your activities since the morning, is in part our natural auto pilot at work when we have fixed routines in our lives. While routines are important for us achieving our goals in life, done mindlessly on auto pilot is known to cause a chronic buildup of stress, boredom and reduces the passion and pleasure of achieving our goals into mundane activities. In a sense mindlessness is ' not living in the present moment'.

What is mindfulness? What is its link to preventing 'Physician burnout"?

Mindfulness has three components; the first component is a state in which one is connected with present moment and aware of their own thought, feelings and sensations internally as well as externally, such that the person is connected to the moment in which he is living. The second component is having a gentle , non-judgmental impression of the internal or external situation that is currently unfolding before the person. And third is intentionally doing what is right and appropriate in a response to the situation, being in line with ones values as discussed in the previous chapter and not being reactive but rather being proactive.

It's in our nature to have a state of mind, in which we worry of the future events or contemplate about the past or dwell on thoughts and emotions, when we are challenged with a difficult or stressful situations. Also, zone out of conscious thinking when we do activities that we are confident with. Either way we are not living in the moment, our awareness is elsewhere and we have not utilized our abilities in that moment.

Example

A good example of mindlessness that exists is in our medical community is, there is a documented evidence of **conformational bias** in experienced physicians.

Experienced doctors can get into trouble by relying on certain treatments with which they had a few prior 'successes'. A practitioner may have once recommended a drug to a patient with certain symptoms. Perhaps that particular patient's symptoms subsided for other reasons, and the patient gave the physician high praise for a job well done. The doctor may continue to recommend this treatment to other patients with similar symptoms. Perhaps a few of them begin to feel better and give the doctor similar praise. The doctor is likely to remember these cases with pride, all the while forgetting the patients that reported no benefit or significant side-effects.

The phrase **"remembering the hits and forgetting the misses"** describes the essence of the confirmation bias.

Skeptical doctors should be cautious not to rely on memorable anecdotes over science.

So is medical experience good? Where does it fail?

A doctor's experience is very helpful, allows picking up on a very subtle symptom early in a disease process, or to determine the right treatment when your condition falls outside of what is taught in textbooks. And for many medical treatments — especially the highly technical ones — there's a direct correlation between physician experience and outcome.

In a variety of situations, though, **experience can backfire**, and the reason is simple psychology. Doctors are human too, and they fall prey to tricks of the mind — like thinking that an ineffective treatment really works due to **conformational bias.** Mental shortcuts can mislead even highly educated, well-seasoned practitioners into making the wrong decisions.

Some intangible benefits to having a "less experienced doctor"

They have a more up-to-date education, enthusiasm and less susceptible to cognitive biases developed by years of practicing and thinking in the same way, the interest to observe the signs and symptoms patiently as there is an innate curiosity to learn and gain experience.

What causes this ?

Over the years of experience, our fixed routines allow our passion for the work we do to become mundane and ordinary sending our brains into auto pilot. We let mindlessness to creep into our lives, due to reliance of on our thoughts from past experiences, and over confidence in our "clinical opinions" that closes the window on the observing present moment completely. It clouds ability to pick up the signs and symptoms in a patient right in front of you, impairing diagnosis, and further management of the patient.

Apart from having consequences in patient health, the consequences for you are higher- Yes Mindlessness is the foundation stone for physicians "professional and emotional burnout."

Mindfulness based stress reduction techniques:

1. A practiced pause

There are thousands of self-help books on communication skills, problem solving skills and they all mention one key component - "the art of listening".

Listening in a MBSR context is the careful attention to the sensations, feelings emotions, thoughts internally as well of others in the external environment .

Step 1. Take a pause.

Amidst a stressful situation, whether its light stress or a panic attack.

a. Being aware of the reality in front of us, without viewing it with prejudice, judgment or strong emotional reactions that we have .

b. Being aware of your of thoughts and emotions and asking questions in a gentle manner :

"Why am I having these thoughts?"

"Are they rational or emotional ?"
"Am I responding in accordance with my values, or am I getting carried away by my emotions ?"

"Am I internalizing someone else's mood, mindset, authority driven fear or white collar bullying?"

c. Being aware of the other persons thoughts

"why is that person acting this way ?"
"what is the reason ?"
"is it rational or irrational ?"
"what is it that the person or situation is demanding of me?"
"what should I do to keep in line with my values of life ?"

d. Intentional action based on "the right thing to do" according to you.

The end result of this technique, is that it helps us be able to focus on reality unaffected by stress and worry and take appropriate decisions in a practical manner that in line with our personal value system. So the stressful situation no longer has the power to affect you.

2. Mindful breathing

Have you noticed after reading for a hour, your body naturally reacts by a need for a small stretch a deep breath and the urge to look around the surrounding to get away from your activity. However short the moment might be it is de-stressing and immensely pleasurable and refreshing.

The essence of this is in the breath. Breath connects you to the present moment, makes you aware of the sensations in your body, the tensions that you are holding in your body due to your reading activity of which you did not notice, as you were so engrossed in the activity . It reconnects you with the environment that you are sitting in, helps you relax your muscles and is a documented MBSR practice. It is known to reduce stress irrespective of the duration of mindful breathing. It can be done for a few seconds at work or during studying or any part of the day to overcome anxieties, stress and worry. It can also be done as meditation during leisure, this practice having its origins in yoga has been scientifically validated.

Technique

Start by moving your attention to the process of breathing. Focus on the sensations of each breath, either focus on the feeling of the movement of air during inhaling and exhaling, at the nostrils. Just observing it as it happens.

As you do this exercise you may find that your mind wanders, you may have thoughts or notice noises in the room, or bodily sensations. On noticing this, know that this is okay, and simply refocus and gently bring your attention back to the breath. This may be performed for a few seconds to as long as time permits.

Apart from stress reduction it can be used to develop, will power, discipline and improved ability to get into the "flow"(a state of intellectual focus) at will .

3. Mindful Eating

Mindful eating helps in stress reduction, maintaining a healthier diet and also has been evidenced to have effects of weight loss. Eating, with awareness of your senses, allow you to enjoy the flavours in a dish. This also allows you to notice when the pleasure from the food starts to decrease.

Eating slowly allows time for the brain to be satisfied and it usually takes 20 minutes for the brain to realize that the stomach is full – allowing you to appreciate quantity over quality.

Because of the attention that you will focus on food and your eating habits you will be able to eliminate bad cravings as you become more aware of the underlying emotions that drive these cravings.

Consistent mindful meditation reduces the amount of stress hormones and cortisol. As we know high cortisol levels are linked to pre-diabetes and obesity. Cortisol also triggers orexins in the body to bring about intense cravings for unhealthy food.

How do you incorporate this into your daily life?

The 2 to 3 minutes to destress when the food is placed before you

Have you ever noticed cravings generally appear when you are stressed. Stress tends to enhance cravings for high caloried comfort foods . To avoid these cravings the next time you are stressed, sit down quietly and maintain good posture. Start to focus on your heart and breathing, breathe deeply and focus your senses on the sensations of inhaling and exhaling. Keep this up for two minutes or more.

Eat mindfully

Start of by eating a one to two meals a day slowly in a quite surrounding and mindfully.

- Remove all distraction (TV, books, technology, phones).
- Savor the look and texture
- Notice the different aromas
- The subtle flavors of every small bite.

- Notice as the taste change and blend within your mouth,
- Only starting the next bite after you have completely eaten the one before.
- You'll notice your bodily sensations shifting, be very aware of this so that you can recognize when you are satisfied and should stop.
- By carrying out mindful eating you start to consume fewer calories and enjoy your food more.

Notice hunger and craving

Try to notice your cravings and hunger that occur at odd times , investigate if the cravings are associated with your emotions

Ask yourself:
"What emotions am I feeling, why am I feeling this way, and what is the best course of action I can take to address this?"

You might realize that you're hungry, or in most other cases that you are fatigued, stressed, or not dealing with other emotions.

Chapter 6

Therapeutic lifestyle choices

We as medical healthcare professionals, advice patients to make therapeutic life choices but it is necessary for us to examine our own lifestyles. We are faced with erratic schedules in our life from the entrance into medical school to the late years of a consultant, which pose a challenge to us, in following therapeutic lifestyle.

There are eight Conner stones of therapeutic lifestyle choices, we need to prioritize in our schedules to prevent burnout in our medical career's and help is build resilience to adverse situations and stress and also help is thrive.

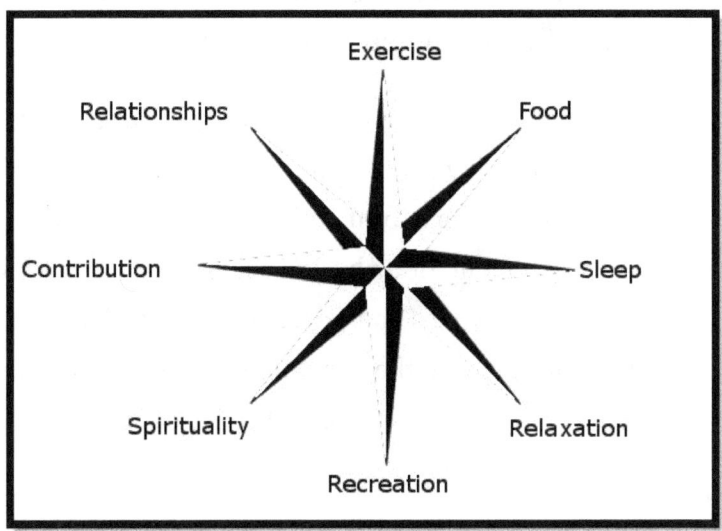

Relaxation:

This book clearly defines the techniques to elicit a relaxation response, the use of mindfulness based practices to guided imagery and progressive muscle relaxation and self-soothing techniques.

Recreation

Recreation is engaging the mind in an activity, that requires sufficient focus on "fun" and enjoyable activities. Its a time to do something, over which you have a sense of control, where you feel competent and empowered, a world where you are in charge.

Whether it is a mental activity such as doing a crossword or painting or drawing (notice the current phenomenon of adult coloring books to beat stress), learning to play a musical instrument, or a physical activity such as running or swimming playing a sport does not matter. The only requirements are that the recreational activity captivates your attention and gives a sense of satisfaction.

Spirituality

Spirituality though less tangible than exercise and sleep is an effective stress tool and is integral to health and wellbeing .Spirituality is not a particular religion or belief system.

Spirituality in context of

- Connecting with yourself and others in the world
- Your personal value system that you live by
- Your search for the greater understanding of life and its purpose

It need not be religion even atheists find a connection with humanity and nature.

The benefits of spirituality as a stress tool

1. Being spiritual is documented to have health benefits, lower cortisol levels, lower inflammatory markers and fewer infections

2. Expanding social reach- For the religious individuals, it could participation in church mosque temple with family or society and for the atheist it could be discussions of the mysteries of the universe explained by pure scientific view

or marveling at the beauty of life humanity or the arts and nature along with likeminded people. Whatever be your definition of spirituality it helps you connect with the world around you.

3. Gives perspective of what is important in our life, defines our values and inspirations and creates a mindset of joy and optimism.

Contribution

Contribution creates a positive mindset as it internally validates your own importance your moral and ethical compass. In any form or magnitude, whether a simple donation to a charity or volunteering for a cause. Even the daily attention you pay to your patients, the ability to empathize be connected and sharing a smile of giving a listening ear knowing that you have made a difference even by a small gesture .Notice that we applaud people in society that have been selfless in society whether its Mother Terrassa or Bill Gates , it doesn't mater if their contribution is for commercial or non-commercial purposes , the bottom line is they have contributed in their own way. They have touched lives and improved society and there is nothing more rewarding psychologically and physiologically, than the work that you do that results in the greater good.

Relationships

Though our close relationships are unconditional, a renewal of our bond on a constant basis is an absolute human requirement. We have evolved as a species as a social being and this dimension of life needs to exist on a daily basis. In the current world we isolate ourselves into mini islands even in a crowd; this does not help our very basic need. Fostering human connection with family or friends or even pleasant small talk with strangers validates our existence in our society.

Over time, loneliness and lack of companionship makes one vulnerable which affects physical and mental health. There has been documented evidence of increased inflammatory makers, cardiac disease and premature death in isolated individuals and mental health issues of depression anxiety and behavioral problems.

Actions we can take:

- Schedule time with family and friends during your day or work week, even if it's a phone call.
- Know that loneliness is just a feeling and not a reality as we can reach out to the world around.

- Be a support to the emotional needs of others, this is an antidote to loneliness.
- Find likeminded people and group activities. Example a study group or morning run group

Exercise:

Thirty minutes of active cardio vascular exercise helps the flow of endorphins ,which help control our stress levels, reduce depression and enhance our memory and cognitive functions. Also, have innumerable effects physiologically in overall fitness, body mass index, and cardiovascular and muscular health which in turn have a positive effect on our mindset.

Food: With scarcity of time and the availability of nutritious choices of food. We must try to preplan meals and make arrangements to consume healthy regular meals, so that we can function well during our stressful week

Sleep:

Sleep is essential cornerstone to stress management, many meta-analyses have shown that sleep has a direct effect on mood, memory consolidation, judgment thus enhancing our personal effectiveness and helping us thrive even in stressful circumstances.

Learning techniques

Learning Techniques

Learning is synonymous with our profession, committing dozens of subjects, different concepts and facts to our memory, is key to our success as doctors. The arduous experience of learning it all over years can bring with it accumulated stress. As we have accepted our rigorous lifestyles of medical education, as part of who we are, we don't give much attention to the stress that successive academic pursuits and our job profiles bring us.

Countless Exams, presentations, the daily volley of questioning at rounds, conferences coupled with clinical work and managing patients, students, professors requires a lot of focused attention and physiologically this stress increases circulating cortisol and catecholamine levels which helps us confront such situations head on .Yet, in the long run can lead to accumulated stress and a burnout . It may impair our ability to learn .Thus learning validated strategies of learning and memory, can help mitigate chronic stress of our academically intensive profession.

Learning & Memory Science

Eminent neuro-scientists and cognitive psychologists have published numerous validated techniques and books .Here is a compilation of six techniques that can be applied to our journey of learning.

Technique 1. Switching between different modes of thinking -"Cut off time"

There are two main modes of thinking, best explained with the analogy of a light beam.

Flood lights at a stadium - akin to a broad thinking pattern.

Laser beam - focused thinking pattern.

These two processes of thinking occur independently in different areas of our brain, both are essential to our learning process.

While focused thinking , helps us in problem solving puts us in a state of attention, and grips our awareness to a point that sometimes we are oblivious to time and our surroundings. This has been idealized by media, self-help books as the ideal state for learning and have come up with techniques to maintain this state for a longer duration.

Contrary to the above, research states that even the diffuse mode is essential to the learning process.

"How?" you may ask.

We are designed for short periods of focused attention. Deliberate focused attention, though helps us rise to challenges, does not help in long term learning. The best example of this is cramming before an exam, helps us raise to the challenge of an assessment but does not help in long term acquisition of skills.

Deliberate focused attention also releases a lot of cortisol and other stress hormones and contributes to rise of inflammatory markers. Pains, aches, headaches, dyspepsia are synonymous with stressful exam.

Broad thinking pattern gives the brain time to process the new found information, make associations to already known information and greatly helps in long term memory and in creativity.

Here a small story to explain the process of how broad mode of thinking works.

On one Sunday morning a doctor was working on a presentation and his 8 year old daughter was rather boisterous singing her rhymes loudly, drumming on the furniture and he was highly distracted .So he took a magazine with a picture of a world map on it , tore it to pieces and gave it to his daughter .He told her to finish the puzzle and tape it back together with all the continents in the right place and when she did he would spend some time with her . In 5 minutes his daughter returned with the puzzle completed, all taped back together.

The doctor was confused, how she managed to do it that fast?

His daughter replied "The mickey mouse picture on the back of the map really helped putting it together ".

If the girl where to have continuous focused attention of solving the puzzle it would have taken her a lot of time ,it was the playful exploration of the girl as to what was on the other side of the puzzle that let her finish the puzzle quickly.

It is in our second nature to make sense of the world around us ,we can remember innumerable names of celebrities , and details of their personal lives , yet studying a complex multi factorial pathophysiology or the mechanism of action of a new drug could be daunting and could take a couple of rounds of reading before it makes sense or permanently committed to memory .

The diffuse mode of thinking gives our brains the ability to associate new ideas with knowledge that we already know.

There are numerous examples of this so called "eureka" moments. Most major scientific breakthroughs, dawning on scientist when they were in the

shower , or taking a walk or having an apple fall on your
head while siting under a tree .

After a session of focused mode of thinking , if one
switches over to the diffuse pattern , by taking a break
and doing something enjoyable (it may be taking a walk
,listening to some music or just mundane things like
cleaning , laundry or chores) helps assimilate the
new information and processes it more rapidly and also
helps in understating it in your own personal manner and
also helps us with problem solving , creativity and finding
innovative solutions to understating new concepts and
daily learning and life problems .

The Technique: "Cut off time"

25 minutes "cut of time "of focused thinking along with 10 minutes of diffuse thinking , is an effective
learning strategy for assimilating new information and committing it to long term memory. Also, helps to avoid procrastination and laziness, with the self-reward of a 10 minute break.

Three hour study period would amount to 1 hour
of leisure activity, which is quite palatable and can help with motivation and assimilate new ideas and accomplish various nonacademic goals simultaneously (like exercise , household chores, drawing, etc. ...)

Technique 2: Recall theory.

There is a overconfidence in our short term working memory.

When we settle down to learn a new chapter or something new, immediately after the study session we have a sense of knowing it and a sense of fulfillment of having assimilated new information, of having understood new concepts. Yet if someone quizzes us on the matter 5 days later without reviewing the content, we would be able to muster up just one or two core concepts but not the finer details. Five months later, definitely not more than 1 core concept.

The explanation:

We have a limited working memory that is bombarded with information all around us, even if you're sitting in a quite library and reading a book, there is information coming to us from all around (it may be the people browsing the aisle or the bright color of a sweater someone wearing, or someone using a new iPad that you

were planning to buy). It's a whole galaxy
of information that you perceive and reading a concept is
just one of them.

We have great ability to understand new concepts, that
gives us a feeling of "learning" but in true sense it's just
perception.

Our brain has a natural tendency to "delete" the unwanted
and non-important experiences from our working memory
, once we are through with that experience . For example :
*could you remember what you had for dinner exactly 2
weeks ago ?*

Likewise sitting in a library and reading a new concept
could also be perceived as unimportant and be
permanently "deleted " and you are more like to remember
the new IPad that your neighbor was using .

Control-S " Saving the experience as a long term memory "

Information of our countless experiences are generally "deleted " , it is only the experiences that contribute to our survival , that have an emotional value is effortlessly ingrained in our memory (an accident, an entertaining movie , a birthday).

How do we remember everyday information like your telephone number or your password to your email?

It's because we have constantly fetched that information from our short term memory (when someone asks for your telephone number , of everyday as you check your email inbox for messages) . The very act of recalling known information, converts short term memory to a long term memory by strengthening the neural pathway.

Studies by cognitive psychologists has showed that the practice of recalling information after a considerable duration post a study session helps " Save " short term memory as long term memory .

Here the catch - Recalling several times on the same day serves no purpose.

Increased duration between recalling
the information helps strengthen the neural pathways more effectively that recalling this many times in a single study session.

The technique "Use mundane activities to "Recall " study sessions"

Long showers, dressing up, household chores or walking are quite ideal to recall the topic that you have studied the previous day.

The very process may seem annoying, you might have the urge to read the book to fill in the gaps of your memory, but wait till you have recalled as much as u can before you do so.

Just like brushing your teeth with your non dominant hand(try it), it's frustrating annoying yet its creating new neural pathways, with a few days of practice you will have the full range of intensity and motion as your dominant hand .Recall to strengthen neural pathways and covert short term memory to long term memory. **"Control S"** **your concepts**.

Technique 3: Go to Sleep.

Now that sounds more like procrastination, but sleep is designed to be our natural playback of all the experiences of the day, the ones that are irrelevant are erased and the ones that have been repeated and held our interest are the ones that are stored in our long term memory.

How can we use this to our advantage?

After a hard day work, or after a day at of lectures and labs for the students, sometimes there is very little energy left to review the things we have learned for the day and the only thing on our minds is to sleep.

Technique: Let your sleep work for you

As you lay there in bed before you go to sleep, mentally recapitulate the information that you want to remember

For example

If it's a particular case that you saw in the wards that you need to remember. Take for instance a rare syndrome or an odd presentation. A quick mental run threw of the case, in terms of the points you want to remember (history , findings on examination lab findings), visualize the signs and what the patient told you and the abnormal lab findings .This can go a long way in retaining the information . Even if u fall asleep midway, its completely acceptable. As your brain recognizes it as an important neural pathway it won't vanish into oblivion like the information from the other experiences of the day like number of red traffic lights on your drive back home, or the color of the clothes that your colleague wore to work . These insignificant pieces of information are deleted . The ones that have been repeated, are considered by your brain to have emotional weightage and value in your survival, are quickly consolidated into long term memories .

There is a lot of truth to the metaphor "Sleep on it"

When faced with a difficult problem or a challenge, remaining in the focused mode of thinking and having a sleepless night does not help in Problem solving. It simply increases your stress levels. Allowing oneself to switch off and move into a broad mode of thinking for a while followed by sleep, can greatly help with problem solving, long term registration of learnt topic and association with well-known ideas and memories.

On revisiting the issue or problem the next morning, the processing of difficult ideas and subjects and problems becomes easier. We can use this technique to commit facts, ideas and concepts to our long term memory.

The few moments before sleep have a profound effect processing of memory. We can use sleep state and dreams akin to tuning our TV'S to a particular channel. Sleep acts as a natural replay to our experiences through the day. We can tune this "playback recorded "to the events that we need to remember.

Method:

After an evening of study sessions, as you turn in to sleep, once the lights are off a quick flash threw of the study session , even if its mere recalling of the names of the categories or subcategories, is enough to tune your mind to process the new information and commit it to long term memory during the sleep cycle.

Technique 4: Association learning: "Our Evolutionary tool box".

It has taken thousands of years for us humans to evolve, the end product is our highly evolved brains. The early humans could scavenge or hunt for food hundreds of miles away from their dwellings and yet make it back to their houses in stormy weather, without maps, roads, signs or GPS. We attribute this quality to our amazing visual special memory. Our highly evolved visual memory can help is remember finer details of the experiences and life situations. As it was essential for our ancestors to survive "Knowing where in the forest the fruits are available, knowing where the lions cave is".

Tool 1: Visual Memory & Imagination.

You can be amazed at how much you can actually remember.

Academics though, revolve around volumes of large stemmed books and assimilating black and white lines. While bestseller fiction authors can manage to create mental images and captivate the mind, reading academic material requires, prior understanding and inherent interest to live up the captivating nature of a bestseller novel.

"This can be evidenced by our increased ability to describe in detail the hero of a novel , compared to   the pathophysiology of Alzheimer disease after just a brief read through of both the these texts ."

Our visual memory is our innate evolutionary tool that we can leverage.

After reading a particular topic that you need to memorize

Step 1. Visualization and imagination

You would need to harness your personal power of creativity to use this method .In clinical subjects create a mental image of a patient with the symptoms of the disease that you are studying, have flowcharts on PowerPoint presentations or charts in your study area.

 This can be applied to basic sciences as well; it's very hard to forget the lipid vacuoles in an adipocyte once you have seen it under a microscope.

Step2. Make it real and tangible - Add details to you mental imagery , give the patient a name ,visualize taking history of the patient and their responses , visualize the signs that you pick up on examination, go to the extent of feeling proud of your ability to diagnose the condition .You can use different types of mental imagery for different subjects .

While studying the histology of adipose tissue, you could probably imagine yourself taking a walk within the cell between the different organelles and structures. Use your creativity to make it tangible and real for yourself. The secret is **the more bizarre you get with the visual analogies the more likely you are to remember it.**

3. Emotional weightage:

If you ask a person to remember his most embarrassing moments he would definably come up with a list in a couple of seconds, yet if u were to ask him something ambiguous as, "can you name the last 10 times that you were very happy?" It would take him quite a while to come you with a list .This can be due to our evolutionally make up of remembering our adverse experiences for the benefit of survival.

For example:

Studying the stages of labor in OB&G , and
imagining doing your first delivery inside a broken lift
where you're the only medical professional around and
being commended in the local newspaper for your quick
action .As bizarre it may seem , would help you remember
all the stages labor much better than only reading it from a
textbook . Create your own scenario for emotional
weightage to the thing that you need to remember.

*"You can't depend on your eyes when your imagination
is out of focus."*

-*Mark Twain*

Tool 2 : Do it yourself - Walking the walk

This is where the idea of clinical rotations comes in , utilizing the experiences that that one comes across in the hospital as learning tool . Understanding the pharmacodynamics of a sympathomimetic drugs can seem incomprehensible to a medical student , with its different actions on different receptors. Yet for an anesthetist it is knowing the back of his palm , his constant use of the drug and observation of its medical effects using his clinical knowledge and monitors , ingrain such information permanently in his long term memory .

"We cannot learn to swim without jumping in the swimming pool " it is essential to give the medical knowledge a tangible and real dimension.

Understating Newton's analogy of gravity as, an apple falling to the ground is simple to comprehend compared to understanding the electro physiology of the heart.

Its only when we correlate knowledge with something tangible in the real word that we truly learning.

Example.

Learning the electro physiology of the heart for a first year medical student is quite difficult compared to an emergency physician, as constant reading of ECG's, gives a tangible real dimension to the pre-existing knowledge .

So, walk the walk.

Exploit opportunities in the clinical rotations to give your theoretical knowledge a tangible dimension.

Tool 3: Mnemonics the good and the bad & why they don't work.

Countless books and websites are dedicated to the use of mnemonics. In many situations though, we can sometimes find it hard to remember the mnemonic itself or maybe remember one or two items in the chain of ideas. There are two reasons behind this

 No personal influence of the mnemonic !! As catchy as it may seem

Lack of consolidating the mnemonic itself into long term memory.

What do we about it?

Make your own mnemonics that have importance in your life

Example :

Usual Mnemonic: to remember the layers of the skin

British and **S**wiss **g**uys **l**ove **c**ornflakes .

B- Basale

S- Spinosum

G- Graulosum

L- lucidum

C- corneum

Seems simple but yet if one were to remember
this mnemonic 3 months later it would be a quite a
challenge.

Now here the technique one needs to add personal
significance to the mnemonic or emotional weightage only
then the mnemonic can be stored in long term memory .

Choose the mnemonic based of your personality , your traits and life experiences .Anything that gives you, personal attachment to it.

For the a fun loving girl -   **C**ome **l**ets **g**o **s**un **b**athing

For the cynical geek   -   **C**ome **l**et's **g**et **sun b**urned

For the Perpetual Romeos- **B**oy **s**ays **g**irl **l**ooks **c**ute

For the dusky   - **B**rown **s**kin **g**otta **l**ook **c**ute

Technique 5: The practice of 'Spaced practice' .

Scientific Background:

Neurosciences have taught us about the concept of "synaptic plasticity", the constant use of a nerve partway helps certain transcription factors to be produced by nerves (Brain derived neurotropic Factor) that cause permanent changes to the nerve structure and function, enhancing the synaptic transmission. The same process help is in converting short term memory to long term memory.

Examples form life.

All of us would have had the traumatic experience of junior school where 'learning the multiplication tables by rote' or 'reciting a famous poetry' would stifled upon us day after day. So let's evaluate what we retain from it now in adulthood? Well we belong to the medical fraternity and we can do these complex multiplications in factions of a second all day long calculating doses of medications based on patients weight and other uses . Yet, if one where to try and recall the list of 3rd grade poetry course, you would probably be able to recite just one or two, despite having recited it every single day at school, during third grade.

The explanation:

The math tables that were recited on a daily basis had a tangible use all though out the person's life at intermittent intervals (We invariably use math multiplications throughout life activities from cooking to calculating a 10 percent tip at the restaurant) thus strengthening the memory .

On the contrary the list of poetry's would only be remembered only if we had an emotional connection with it or considered it a favorite , thus a person would remember just a handful of the entire course of third grade poetry class

The Method:

Spaced repetition is the best way to convert short term memory to long term memory and can be used to enhance ones learning skills.

If one where to learn some new topic , the text material needs to be read repeatedly **NOT on the same day** at intervals as suggested, in the table below.

Example:

Day 1	Day 2	Day 5	Day 7	Day 10	Day 14
Topic 1	Topic 1	Topic 1	Topic 1	Topic 1	Topic 1

The above will be an ideal example of a spaced practice schedule, to learn and assimilate new information pertaining to one single topic.

Technique 6: Interleaving.

In a continuation from Spaced practice, interleaving as the name suggests involves having multiple topics to rotate in a single study session.

Day 1	Day 2	Day3	Day4	Day 5
Topic 1	Topic1	Topic5	Topic5	Topic4
Topic2	Topic3	Topic6	Topic7	Topic2
Topic3	Topic2	Topic7	Topic6	Topic1
Topic4	Topic4	Topic8	Topic8	Topic3

In the table above the topics have been interleaved each of the 4 days, they have also been spaced out during the week as specified in the chapter of spacing.

A combination of interleaving and spacing is most effective.

Technique 7: Exercise.

Our physiology has a lot to do with the adequate functioning of our brain, Processes of memory and learning.

Various cognitive scientists have documented that exercise boots learning capacity and memory.

The Exercise for this module is to exercise

A brisk walk or a sprinting, asana's from yoga or Pilates choose your weapon of choice and follow through, preferably outdoors as the sights & sounds of outdoor exercise is known to help with association learning.

www.lifehacksfordoctors.org

Coming soon:

Time Management skills for doctors